HORMONE RESET

BALANCE YOUR HORMONES, START THE WEIGHT LOSS JOURNEY, GET 50+ EXICITING HORMONE RESET DIET RECIPES

Introduction

When trying to lose weight, many ideas might come up, ranging from exercise, dietary changes and lifestyle changes. Sometimes you will get everything right and still find yourself gaining some weight. Weight loss is a factor of the interaction of various hormones that determine how the body utilizes food taken by the body.

With hormonal imbalance it, not only weight gain that you will experience, but you might experience other symptoms. Low levels of energy, fatigue, irregular periods, high blood pressure, and memory loss may sometimes be an indicator of hormonal imbalance. This book breaks down various hormones that will affect your weight, their symptoms, and a guide on how to reset these hormones.

The hormone reset diet will give you various foods that will keep your hormones in balance as you begin your weight loss journey and breakdown the differences between hormone imbalance in women and men.

I. Thyroid Hormones

These are hormones in the blood that are produced by a part of the body known as the thyroid gland, which is found around the neck. These hormones are available to the body through the consumption of food with iodine.

Thyroid hormones have several roles in the body. They are essential when it comes to basal metabolic rate, long bone growth, neural maturation, and protein synthesis. They are also responsible when it comes to increasing body sensitivity during the intake of chemicals like catecholamine, for instance, adrenaline. All cells in a human being's body depend on these hormones when it comes to their differentiation and development. In relation to the weight gain of a human body, the hormones act as regulators in the metabolism of fats, proteins, and carbohydrates. It is their role to control the usage of energy compounds within a human's body cells. At the same time, the hormones are useful in stimulating the metabolism of vitamins. When there is an increase in the hormones, the body tends to facilitate an increase in the weight of the patient, and sometime he may end up becoming obese. However, a decrease in the hormones happens to be causing an urge to consume a lot of food. Unfortunately, the metabolism is affected, and the person instead loses weight despite high food consumption.

Symptoms

Some of the significant signs that are relative to the thyroid hormone imbalance are as following;

- The person may experience dryness or coarse skin and hair.
- There is also a tendency to be forgetful.
- Signs of exhaustion and fatigue are prevalent.
- Due to the swelling of the thyroid gland, the person will develop a hoarse voice.
- Depending on the hormone imbalance, the person will experience weight gain or loss. It is important to note that not all weight conditions are due to thyroid hormones imbalance.
- Women happen tendency of irregular menstrual. It is also essential to get medical counsel before concluding that the hormones are lacking.
- In some cases, the person affected may have a form of intolerance to cold.
- At some situation, there is an enlargement of the thyroid gland, which is commonly known as goitre.

Resetting the hormone

- Avoid various varieties of millet, processed foods from wheat and un-prescribed supplements.
- Some foods should be taken in moderation, such as soy foods, foods with gluten such as wheat, bulgur, and graham flour among others.
- Reduce the consumption of cruciferous vegetables such as Broccoli, Brussels sprout, Cabbage and Cauliflower among very many others in this category
- Eat foods rich in selenium, iodine and zinc such as Brazilian nuts, eggs, all types of meat – whether red or white meat – seafood including the likes of salmon, tuna and shrimp.
- Smoking has been known to cause different types of hormone imbalance so you might have to go slow on the butts
- Eat more foods with antioxidants such as eggplant, berries, grapes, apricots, spinach , red wine, tea, sea food and lean meat among others
- Reduce the amount of sugar in your diet, sugar can easily cause inflammation in the body slowing down the conversion of T4 to triiodothyronine
- Take foods rich in vitamin B-12 such as peas, asparagus, sesame seeds, tuna, cheese, milk and eggs
- Take foods rich in Probiotics such as yoghurt, raw cheese, kefir, kombucha, kimch and sourdough bread.
- Get enough sleep, 8 hours sleep is recommended
- Engage in less physical exercises and yoga

https://www.medicinenet.com/script/main/art.asp?articlekey=38373
https://www.empoweryourhealth.org/magazine/vol7_issue1/the_thyroid_hormones_and_body_weight_issues
https://www.healthline.com/nutrition/hypothyroidism-diet#section3

II.   Cortisol Hormone

Cortisol hormone belongs to a class of hormones that are responsible in glucose regulation in the blood. It has been found to offer effectiveness in controlling the salt and water in the body in order to maintain a balance state of these two.

The purpose of this hormone to the body is to help in reducing inflammation, regulate metabolism, control sugar levels and aids in memory formulation. Due to these functions, the hormone is a crucial part in the body helping it to maintain a balanced weight.

Most of the time, cortisol hormone has been related as a stress hormone. Although this may be one of the factor, it is more of adrenaline related hormone. In that case, when a part of the body known as adrenal glands detect some changes in the level of body adrenaline, they happen to send a signal to the body that results to an effect on cortisol levels.

Cortisol levels changes either in increase or in decrease. Either changes in level affect the blood sugar levels. In turn, at a high level the body happens to gain weight at a higher potential and when they lower, the body losses its weight more than anticipated.

Symptoms

Whether at a high or lower levels, cortisol changes may lead so several notable symptoms.

- A rapid increase in weight especially around the chest, face and the abdomen which is un-proportional to legs and arms.
- Tiredness that is very unrealistic.
- One may experience dizziness especially when standing.
- When the face is round and flushed then there is a change on the hormone change.
- Weight loss especially upon lower levels.
- High blood pressure is another symptom.
- The skin becomes sensitive, darkens and get bruises plus purple like stretch marks.
- One develops weakness in relation to the muscles.
- Depression, irritability and anxiety that are incorporated to moody circumstances.
- Lacking or unsatisfactory sleep.
- An increase in the frequency of urination and an increased thirst.

Hormone Reset

- ➤ Avoid meals and beverages that have processed sugar and unsafe fats so that to manage blood sugar such as white sugar, caffeine, sodas, white flour, fast food, alcohol, processed food and artificial sweeteners.
- ➤ Cortisol hormone level is known to spike during stressful moments and go down after the stress is over, but when you are constantly under stress the levels will stay high.
- ➤ Get enough rest and sleep
- ➤ Avoid caffeine and alcohol before bed
- ➤ If possible take early morning exercises as opposed to afternoon exercise and also you might have to consider yoga and Pilates as opposed to more physical workouts.
- ➤ Take foods rich in omega 3 such as mackerel, oysters, sardines, salmon, Herring, Anchovies, flaxseeds, chia seeds, walnuts, soybeans, among others
- ➤ Take foods rich in vitamin C found in most fruits and vegetables
- ➤ Take foods rich in vitamin B5

https://www.hormone.org/your-health-and-hormones/glands-and-hormones-a-to-z/hormones/cortisol
https://www.healthline.com/health/adrenal-fatigue-diet#outlook
https://www.healthline.com/nutrition/12-omega-3-rich-foods#section13

III. Estrogen Hormone

Estrogen is one of the main sex hormone found in women in a more significant proportion than in men. In this category of hormones, there is progesterone which will be discussed later. Its manifestation is in a females' physical appearances and their reproduction system.

Role on the Body and Weight

Estrogen's signs are much clearer during puberty when a girl undergoes changes that brings her transformation into a woman. They include the changes in her physical features like breasts and heaps, growing of pubic and underarm hair, and the beginning of menstrual cycles. Besides, a women's reproductive system and menstrual cycle are controlled by this hormone. Other roles in the body include the controlling of bone development and health for both male and female, brain stability during moods, heart operation, skin and other tissues development. At the same time, it is responsible for keeping check of human cholesterol hence balancing a woman's weight gain.

Cause of Imbalance

Like any other hormone, the body may either have estrogen in smaller or larger quantity. The leading factor to an imbalance in estrogen has been understood to be birth control pills or the initiated estrogen replacement. It is also common to find an imbalance due to the kind of diet one takes. Women also experience a low estrogen production when they reach menopause or when they undergo ovaries' removal surgery. Dietary causes include excessive consumption of cruciferous vegetables which reduce high estrogen levels but may be used when one has too much estrogen. Consuming factory farmed products can also raise estrogen levels. It's a common practice for farms to use hormones such as testosterone, acetate and progesterone among others. When used, this hormones have the ability to cause imbalance to several hormones including estrogen.

Effect on Weight

Estrogen hormone imbalance is more on the lower side than on the increase apart from during a girl's development stage of puberty. In line with this, women are found to gain more weight whenever the hormone lowers. Although a woman body weight gain is typical to the hips and breast, estrogen lowering leads to un-comparative body weight gain, especially in the belly and the thighs.

Symptoms

When the estrogens are lower in the body, woman may experience the following;

- Unbalanced or no menstrual periods.
- Irregular hot flashes plus night sweats.
- Having sleeplessness at night.
- The vagina may become drier and thinner.
- The desire for sex is decreased.
- An extreme headache and menstrual migraine before the periods.
- One becomes moody.
- The skin becomes drier.

- Men may have low desire for sex and additional belly fat.

On the other hand, a high level of estrogen may be factored out through these symptoms.

- Weight gaining.
- Menstrual disorder such as heavy or lower bleeding.
- The premenstrual syndromes are usually heightened.
- Having some lumps on the breasts that are noncancerous.
- Noncancerous fibroid within the uterus.
- Signs of too much exhaustion despite little work.
- Losing sexual desire for men and women.
- Anxiety and signs of depression.
- Men may have abnormal breast enlargement, infertility, and even weaker erections.

Hormone reset

- ➢ Avoid alcohol during the reset period except for a glass or half glass of red wine once in while at dinner accompanied by light snacks such as peanuts.
- ➢ Check the details of any meat product you consume otherwise minimise meat consumption and increase intake of healthy proteins
- ➢ Increase fiber intake in your diet from fruits, vegetables and nuts
- ➢ Avoid unhealthy fats found in processed foods and take more monosaturated fats as a substitute found in nuts, avocado, canola oil, olive oil, sunflower oil, peanut oil and butter and sesame oil

https://www.hormone.org/your-health-and-hormones/glands-and-hormones-a-to-z/hormones/estrogen
https://flo.health/menstrual-cycle/menopause/symptoms/estrogen-rich-foods
https://www.medicalnewstoday.com/articles/321837.php

IV.   Insulin Hormone

The cells get glucose from the blood for them to have the energy required to function correctly. The hormone responsible for making this possible is known as insulin. Insulin comes from the food and is processed by an internal organ known as pancreas found behind a humans stomach. It is then transferred to the body and is produced in accordance with the need relative to glucose level in the blood.

Role on the Body and Weight

The primary purpose is to balance the sugar levels in the blood, and therefore it is produced more if the level of sugars in the blood is high. At the same time, when the blood transfers proteins and fats, it is the responsibility of insulin to break them down into the amount reliable for the body. Apart from breaking sugars from carbohydrates, it is also responsible for the storage of glucose that the body may need to use in the future. This happens to cover for situations when the sugars in the blood cells are lower.

Cause of Imbalance

An imbalance in insulin is considered when the sugar levels are higher than the insulin or otherwise. Some of the inequality occurs due to the individual's weight, especially when one is overweight or obese. Another cause of imbalance would be the intake of too many carbohydrates and sugars, habitual steroids overdose, or a medical condition such as polycystic ovary disease in women.

Effect on Weight

When there is insulin resistance in the body, there is an addition of body weight. Coincidentally, insulin turns out to be proper storage for fats, especially around the belly and so an individual stands a chance of body weight addition. Within a short period, one discovers that he or she has a situation of gaining unexplained weight.

Symptoms

Most of the insulin resistance is triggered by a combination of different facts, including age, weight, and genes. In turn, one may experience the following symptoms.

- Situations of excessive sweating.
- One can develop a larger waist due to fatty berries.
- Some difficulties while sleeping.
- The sensitivity to cold and heat is affected.
- Metabolism is affected.
- There could be changes that are related to the heart rate.
- In some circumstances, an individual develops dark patches and skin rashes.
- In some situation, the heart blood pressure is affected.

Dietary Recommendation

- Limit sugar intake to 15g per day. Any snack should have nutritional values attached to it so the next time you buy a soft drink or ice-cream kindly check the nutritional information
- When taking food, reduce the portion size to avoid excess calories than needed by the body since this excess calories will end up being stored as fats around your belly.
- Be active, physical inactivity leads to low energy expenditure
- Reduce the amount of carbohydrates in your diet
- Consume a lot of soluble fibre found in legumes, fruits, vegetables and some nuts
- Take some green tea
- Use sugar processed sugar substitutes such honey, stevia, agave nectar and coconut sugar among others
- Add cinnamon to food and beverages
- Add some apple and cider vinegar to your diet
- Engage in exercises that can help you lose belly fat

➢ Consider fatty fish in your diet like salmon, sardines, mackerel, herring and anchovies

https://www.medicalnewstoday.com/articles/323760.php
https://health.clevelandclinic.org/polycystic-ovary-syndrome-pill-not-remedy/

V.   Leptin Hormone

What Is The Hormone?

Leptin is a hormone found in the part of the blood known as adipose. It coordinates with the brain part referred to as hypothalamus to send relevant signals during food intake.

Role on the Body and Weight

The hormone is essential for the body since its main purpose is to inform the body when one is satisfied to eat. It facilitates sending of a signal to the digestive system that one has a full stomach. In turn, one can regulate the amount of food consumed during an instance. Therefore, it is responsible for keeping the body at the watch of the food that is enough as per the body mass ratio. Due to its trigger when eating, one can only eat that which is enough and so one cannot add weight unnecessarily.

Cause of Imbalance

An imbalance of leptin is mostly caused by too much sugar consumption. The leading food with a lot of sugar is those that are highly processed and modified since they have more fructose. The product consumption allows fat production, and it is a secreting agent to leptin.

Effect on Weight

An imbalance of this hormone is the leading factor to one consuming a lot of food that the body does not need. In turn, there are high chances that the body will process more food to the body system. As a result, that which will not be used will be deposited as fat in the body hence an increase in body weight.

Symptoms

An imbalanced Leptin hormone can lead to an unhealthy lifestyle which will be detected by different symptoms such as;

- Weight addition that cannot be well explained.
- Excessive food cravings, especially sugary foods.
- Uncontrollable sweating cycles.

- One get stressed, and sleeping becomes difficult and unusual.
- When taking food, one never eats enough as needed.
- Disliking traditional food and only wanting modern diets.
- One develops high blood pressure.

Hormone reset

- Consume healthy fats and proteins in the morning which allows the body to have building blocks for the hormones
- Eliminate and sugar from your diet
- Limit the amount of processed foods you take
- Avoid snacking which will often lead to food cravings and reduce cravings use octane oil as well as coconut oil
- Eat early, give yourself around 4 hours after eating and before sleep
- Time your work outs well, the work outs should never an hour before or after breakfast

https://www.stylecraze.com/articles/hormones-responsible-for-weight-gain-in-women/#gref
https://www.healthline.com/nutrition/leptin-101
https://www.hormone.org/your-health-and-hormones/glands-and-hormones-a-to-z/hormones/leptin

VI.   Ghrelin Hormone

This hormone found and released by the stomach and in small quantity within the small intestine. It is also known as the appetite stimulator or a hunger hormone.

Role on the Body and Weight

The purpose of the hormone is to trigger that one is hungry and also responsible for making sure that depositing of fat is done effectively. It works with the body in the blood cells and the brain to pass on this internal body communication. In small proportion, the hormone is also responsible for triggering the brain when it comes to the rewarding process. Most importantly, the hormone facilitates growth so that the body is able to break fats and can facilitate the building of muscles. It is partially responsible when it comes to the release of insulin in the bloodstream. For that reason, when the hormone is moderate in the bloodstream, it allows the body to balance the amount of body weight.

Cause of Imbalance

The imbalance of the hormone comes about depending on the food intake. When one is taking food, the hormone is at a lower level while one is hungry and even fasting, the ghrelin hormone is at a rise. Some known disorders include prader willi syndrome, cachexia and anorexia nervosa

Effect on Weight

When there are high levels of this hormone in the body, the body tends to add weight more than normal due to the continuous urge to eat.

Symptoms

Ghrelin hormone is much related to eating habits, and most signs are only observed in relation to a person's food consumption. They include;

- Extreme hunger is a common factor.
- Rapid weight addition.
- There is a tendency of weak bones.
- Big craving for sugary things, especially in processed food.
- Unstable thinking trend and memory problems.
- Stress and depression.
- One experiences tiredness yet cannot get enough sleep.

Hormone reset

- ➤ Avoid sugar and sugar products and high fructose foods and drinks that lead to the impairment of ghrelin response after meals leading to reduced satiety feeling.
- ➤ Make sure you include proteins in every meal including breakfast which reduce ghrelin levels and bring about satiety feeling

https://www.ncbi.nlm.nih.gov/pmc/articles/PMC3060653/

VII.   Testosterone Hormone

Just like women have oestrogen as the main sex hormone, men have testosterone as a sex hormone. The fertility, muscle development, red blood cell production, and fat distribution in a man depends highly on the proper functioning and stability in this hormone. It is produced by the brain in conjunction with a body part known as pituitary gland before being released to the blood cells.

Role on the Body and Weight

The hormone is responsible for giving men strength in the bones, to burn fats and to strengthen the muscles. Their libido is also improved by the stability of testosterone hormones. In addition, we find that the bone mass of a man, muscle sizing to the adequate level, fat distribution, and the production of red blood cell in a man entirely depend on this hormone. The roles are also common in a woman, although it is not the dominant one for them with an adequate level of this hormone, a man's weight is stabilized since it is well regulated.

Cause of Imbalance

Aging in a man is the main factor that makes the testosterone to lower in the body. However, it may be because the person has contracted a disease that affects the hormones balance, and this can be controlled through the administration of remedies such as prohormone supplements. It is important to know that the supplements may not work when the imbalance is due to aging.

Effect on Weight

When the testosterone is high, the body happens to add more weight, but when lowered, it reduces the weight and even acts as an agent to the burning of more calories.

Symptoms

Men may experience a variety of levels of testosterone and notice this due to several symptoms.

- Their sexual drive is affected.
- There is an increase in weight and body fats.
- They end up with a dysfunctional erection.
- The sperm count is lower than average.
- Breast tissues may become larger than usual.
- Women get affected by changed body shape, and the size of their breasts reduces.
- Women develop oily skin, and the facial hair grows around the body, the chin, and the lips.

- There can be a loss of strength, and muscle development is not normal.

  Hormone Reset

  ➢ The recommended foods include Tuna, low fat milk, egg yolks, fortified cereals, oysters, shellfish, beans and beef.

  ➢ Sleep is essential in any hormones production and so is testosterone this is backed by comprehensive research

  ➢ Other weight loss strategies such as exercise should be considered for quick results

  ➢ Stress reduction is also major boost to testosterone production

  ➢ Alcohol and drug abuse should be avoided

https://www.medicalnewstoday.com/articles/276013.php

https://www.yourhormones.info/hormones/testosterone/

https://www.hormone.org/your-health-and-hormones/glands-and-hormones-a-to-z/hormones/testosterone

VIII. Progesterone Hormone

The hormone is found in women and is in the reproduction system and mostly manifested during the menstrual cycle, embryogenesis, and pregnancy. It is categorized in a group of hormones known as steroids or progestogens making it a major one in these hormones.

Role on the Body and Weight

The primary role has been to allow a woman to have a regular menstrual cycle and to have safe early pregnancy stages. It researched that it is responsible for giving the body the signals that a woman's body is ready for pregnancy whenever the egg is fertilized. It is also a facilitating factor in giving feedback whenever the egg is not fertilized to initiate another menstrual cycle. It will also take charge in preparation of the body during the early stages of pregnancy and later for childbearing.

Cause of Imbalance

The hormone is manifested at a higher level during the menstrual periods and when a woman is pregnant. As a result, this makes them the only triggers for its high level since later it lowers.

However, it has always been noted to remain higher, especially when a woman takes birth control pills.

Effect on Weight

When its heightening is caused by the contraceptives, the woman has a tendency of increasing their weights. It is normally possible to find that a woman during pregnancy adds more weight since the hormone is produced at a higher level than usual. Nevertheless, when the imbalance is at the lower side, the woman still adds weight since estrogen is left dominant, leading to higher weight addition.

Symptoms

Most side effects of this hormone are when it is at a lower level and apart from weight gaining the symptoms include;

- Trouble becoming pregnant or the pregnancy is not prolonged.
- There situations of headaches or migraines.
- One becomes moody to the extent of anxiety and depression.
- The menstrual cycles are affected and become irregular, absent, or abnormal uterine bleeding.
- Sexual drive is affected by the decreased situation.
- The breasts become tender and may become fibrocystic.
- The gallbladder may develop some problems.

Hormone Reset

➤ Increase intake of vitamins B and C contained in fruits, meat, eggs, dairy products, legumes seeds and nuts among others

➤ Increase intake in foods that contain zinc especially shellfish which is low calories source

➤ Stress contributes to the imbalance therefore stress reduction is way towards progesterone balance

https://www.yourhormones.info/hormones/progesterone/

https://www.webmd.com/vitamins/ai/ingredientmono-760/progesterone

https://www.healthline.com/health/womens-health/low-progesterone#progesterone-levels

IX.   Melatonin Hormone

The Melatonin hormone is one of the hormones that are natural in the body and is made available through one of the glands known as pineal glands. The hormone is very active at night and elevated for the 12 hours when it is dark and then its start levelling back lower as the day unwinds at around 9 am. It is barely impossible to detect its levels during the day.

Role on the Body and Weight

It is the hormone responsible for regulating the time one sleeps and rises up. For this reason, it is responsible when it comes to refreshing one's body. The hormone is also made more effective due to the darkness so that it also facilitates the body's growth. Therefore, it is important to highlight that this hormone is in charge of improving the body's composition, the healing process, the building of lean muscles, and the increasing of bone's density. When in good balance, one is able to maintain body weight since it is capable of moderating various metabolic hormones in charge of how bod works.

Cause of Imbalance

The body has been built to have a stable state whether the hormone is naturally high or low. Its high state is triggered by the darkness, and the opposite is during the day. However, due to medication, induced methods are responsible for taking melatonin higher than the normal state, which may lead to an imbalance.

Effect on Weight

Whenever the hormone is working correctly, the body will be able to control the weight through moderating hormones that regulate satiety, appetite, calorie uptake, and the storage of fats in the body. When the hormone is controlled by medicine, it means all these factors will be affected, and in turn, there will be weight gaining.

Symptoms

Several side effects have been noted whenever there is a high dosage of administered melatonin hormone.

- Drowsiness and the body temperature is lower than usual.
- One may have some headaches during the day.
- One experiences some moments of agitation or nausea.
- Undesired sleepiness which is sometimes intentional but may be unnecessary during the day.
- Short term depression situations.

- At times one gets stomach cramps and a heightened irritation.
- Excessive bleeding, especially for those who have the disorder.
- The risk of having a seizure is heightened.
- Blood pressure is raised, especially for people who already medical situation and need to control the blood pressure.

Melatonin Hormone reset

> Increase consumption of dairy products, poultry products, seafood such as shrimp, salmon, halibut, and tuna and cod which contain Tryptophan which when ingested are converted into neurotransmitter serotonin and later into melatonin
> Nuts and seeds such as pumpkins, sunflower, cashew nuts, peanuts among others also contain tryptophan
> Some legumes contain tryptophan such as chickpeas, black beans, split peas, kidney beans and lima beans.
> Fruits also contain tryptophan for instance bananas, avocado, apples and also vegetables such as spinach, turnip greens, asparagus and seaweed.
> Some grains such as corn, oats, and barley contain Tryptophan

https://www.webmd.com/vitamins/ai/ingredientmono-940/melatonin

https://www.yourhormones.info/hormones/melatonin/

https://www.healthline.com/nutrition/melatonin-side-effects#section8

X.   Glucocorticoid Hormones

The hormone is common in the body since it is categorized as a steroid hormone that the body makes from cells found in zona fasciculata. It has the capacity to send signals to the body for the sake of immunity.

Role on the Body and Weight

The hormone is the leading agent in the body when it comes to reducing the inflammation. It is the same hormone responsible for reducing how sugars or glucose are broken and utilized in the body system as energy. The way fats, sugar, and proteins are needed and broken down in the body is controlled by glucocorticoids hormones. When they are all well regulated, the body is also able to regulate and balance the weight.

Cause of Imbalance

The only reason that has been proven to be a leading reason for a glucocorticoid's imbalance is due to sickness. One of the known illness has been identified as Cushing disease named scientifically as hyperadrenocorticism. Unfortunately, another increasing reason for the imbalance is usually overdose and misuse of drugs with a glucocorticoid as a major agent.

Effect on Weight

When glucocorticoids are in excess in the body, the person exhibits weight addition situations and maintained obesity is a very high possibility. In addition, bodyweight increases at a rate higher than the normal circumstance. When it is lower in the body, there are chances of the individual losing weight at a rapid abnormal rate.

Symptoms

The obvious symptom of imbalance of this hormone is weight addition. Others include;

- Shoulder become fatty and humpy.
- The face may become round.
- Getting some pin stretch marks.
- The bones get weaker too.
- Diabetes and high blood pressure become common.
- The skin becomes thinner, causing a delayed healing process.
- Women happen to exhibit situations of irregular menstrual cycles.
- There is a high rate of fatigue and possibilities of decreased libido.
- Depression and stress become a common factor.

Hormone Reset

➢ Increase intake of foods with vitamin D

https://hopes.stanford.edu/glucocorticoids/
http://www.vivo.colostate.edu/hbooks/pathphys/endocrine/adrenal/gluco.html
https://www.healthline.com/health/glucocorticoids#side-effects

BREAKFAST
ZERO BELLY OMELET

Nutrition

Servings 1
Calorie 226
Protein 17g
Fat 14g
Fiber 2g

Ingredients

- 1 large Portobello mushroom cap
- ½ tablespoon olive oil, divided
- 1 egg
- 2 egg whites
- 1/8 avocado
- Salt and pepper to taste
- Herbs and spices, your choices

Preparation

i. Switch on the broiler and preheat it in advance. Taking a large baking sheet and line it with foil.

ii. Get rid of the mushroom stem first. Take the mushroom cap and brush with half of the olive oil and use salt by sprinkling some on top and place it on the baking sheet with the grilled side facing up. Use the broiler for cooking the mushroom for 5 minutes until it is soft.

iii. Take the remaining oil and heat it over a non-stick pan on medium-low heat. Pour the egg and the egg white in a bowl and whisk then cook it on the pan until the egg sets before removing from the heat.

iv. Take the mushroom and top it with the eggs and the sliced avocado. Use some more salt, pepper to season and your choice of herbs and natural spices.

https://www.mensjournal.com/food-drink/12-zero-belly-recipes/

MEXICAN HORCHATA
Nutrition
Servings 7Cups

Calorie 322
Carbohydrate 56g
Protein 6g
Fat 7g
Fiber 0g

Ingredients

- 1 cup of white rice
- 1 1/3 cup sugar
- ½ cup chopped almonds
- 1 cinnamon stick
- 1 T vanilla
- 1 can (12 ounces) evaporated milk
- 1 ½ cup of milk, almond milk
- 1 liter of water
- Ice

Preparation

i. Soak first the rice, cinnamon, and almonds in a bowl with water for the night or 5 hours earlier before the preparation time.

ii. When starting the preparation, you can drain and dispose of the water that was earlier soaked.

iii. Put the mixture in a blender then add evaporated milk and blend until the mixture has wholly formed a smoother combination. Ensure that the rice grains are thoroughly grounded.

iv. Pour the mixture into a pitcher where you will add sugar, vanilla, and the almond milk. Stir to combine the additional ingredients with the blended ones. Add the water and continue stirring.

v. You can use the ice during the serving and enjoy the smoothie.

https://www.mylatinatable.com/authentic-horchata-recipe/

BLACK BEAN BROWNIE BATTER

Nutrition
Servings 42
Calorie 26
Carbohydrate 4.1g
Protein 1g
Fat 0.8g
Cholesterol 0mg
Fiber 0.6g
Sugar 1.6g

Ingredients

- 1 can chickpeas/black beans
- 2 tablespoons regular cocoa powder
- ½ cup quick oats
- ¼ teaspoon salt
- 1/3 cup sweetener of choice
- Pinch uncut stevia
- 2 teaspoon pure vanilla extract
- ¼ cup nut butter
- Chocolate chips
- Milk of choice

Preparation

i. Excluding the add-ins, take the rest of the ingredients, put in the food processor and blend them thoroughly until they are smooth.
ii. Take the chocolate chips and stir inside the solution.
iii. Serve with the add-ins on the side and enjoy for breakfast.

https://chocolatecoveredkatie.com/2017/05/29/dark-chocolate-brownie-batter-dip/

BANANA OAT FLAPJACKS

Nutrition

Servings 8
Calorie 119
Carbohydrate 18.2g
Protein 2.4g
Fat 4.3g
Fiber 1.5g
Sugar 10g

Ingredients

- 50g flaked almonds, toasted
- 150g rolled oats
- 90g self-raising flour
- 50g dried apricots, chopped
- 70g soft brown sugar
- 125g low-fat spread, melted
- 3 tablespoon golden syrup
- 2 medium-ripe bananas, mashed
- 2 teaspoon vanilla extract

- 1 egg

Preparation

i. Switch on the oven and turn the heater to 180 degrees Celsius. Take a baking tin and grease then line it with a baking paper.

ii. Take the dry ingredients, put in a mixing bowl and then take the spread, syrup, vanilla, eggs and smashed bananas and stir to combine them well. Transfer the mixture into the pre-prepared tin.

iii. Place them into the oven and allow them to bake for 20 to 25 minutes or until you can see the light golden brown. Then you touch, and it is firm, then it has cooked. Take the meal out of the cooker and let it cool down first.

iv. After it has rested and cooled for 10 minutes, you can slice into squares and leave it to continue cooling down completely.

v. The flapjacks are ready to be served.

https://www.deliciousmagazine.co.uk/recipes/banana-oat-flapjacks/

BRUSCHETTA WITH MUSHROOM & FONTINA

Nutrition

Servings 8
Calorie 185
Carbohydrate 17g
Protein 7g
Fat 10g
Fiber 1g
Sodium 305mg

Ingredients

- 3 tablespoons extra virgin olive oil
- 10 ounces of Cremini mushrooms, thinly sliced
- 2 sprigs fresh mint
- 2 tablespoon finely chopped shallot
- 1 clove garlic, finely chopped
- 1/2cup hearty red wine, such as Chianti
- 4 wide slices crusty bread, about 8 inches across
- 1cupp shredded Fontina cheese,
- 2 sprigs fresh thyme, plus more for garnish
- Seas salt
- Freshly black pepper, grounded

Preparation

i. Heat the oven's broiler to a high heat level while the rack is positioned 6 inches from the broiler's heating source. On a large skillet, pour 2 tablespoons of the olive oil and heat when it is on medium-high hot.

ii. Place the mushrooms, mint and thyme into the skillet and cook while stirring making sure that they lose their juice and begins to turn brownish; that is for about 6 minutes. Add to the mushrooms the shallot, garlic and cook while occasionally stirring for another 2 minutes until they are tender.

iii. Take the wine and pour to the meal and cook for another 2 minutes so that it is almost reduced then add salt and pepper to taste before removing from the heat; make sure you keep them warm.

iv. Drizzle the bread on the baking sheet and 1 tablespoon of the oil. Let the bread toast in the broiler for about 1 minute then turn and allow it to cook for another 30 seconds, Take the cheese and divide it over the bread before broiling for another 1 minute until it turns brown and crusty.

v. Take the bread from the oven and take the mushroom mixture and discard the herb sprigs. Serve in portions on the bread you prepared from the oven.

vi. Slice each of the bread vertically into half, and you may use some fresh sprigs to the top while serving serve.

https://www.goodhousekeeping.com/food-recipes/easy/a46632/bruschetta-with-mushrooms-and-fontina/

MATCHA GREEN TEA SORBET
Nutrition
Servings 4
Calorie 129
Carbohydrate 33g
Protein 0g
Fat 0g

Ingredients
- 1 tablespoon matcha/green tea powder
- 2/3 cup granulated sugar
- 2 cups water

Preparation
i. Pick a bowl and pour both the green tea and sugar and mix to combine.

ii. Take water portioned and pour in a saucepan and add the mixture then heat until the sugar has dissolved completely.

iii. Remove the pan and place it over a large bowl of water to cool it down until it attains the room temperature.

iv.   Pour the solution into a container that can be used in the freezer and transfer to cool it down. After 30 minutes, you can stir it then leave it to freeze to the almost frozen point.

v.   Remove from the freezer, serve it in glasses, and enjoy.

https://www.thespruceeats.com/matcha-green-tea-sorbet-recipe-2031122

CHILLED CUCUMBER, DILL AND YOGURT

Nutrition

Servings 4

Calorie 316

Carbohydrate 8.9g

Protein 13.6g

Fat 24.8g

Fiber 1.6g

Sugar 8g

Salt 0.8g

Ingredients

- 500g Greek yogurt
- 2 cucumbers
- 1 garlic clove, sliced
- 1 small bunch mint, leaves picked
- 1 small bunch dill
- 2 tablespoons white wine vinegar
- 1 ½ teaspoon celery seeds
- White pepper
- 100g feta, finely crumbled
- 1-2 tablespoons extra-virgin oil
- Rye bread, thinly sliced, to serve

Preparation

i.   Pour the yogurt into a blender. On the side, deseed the cucumber and reserve a little peace and the seeds.

ii.   Chop the cucumber into small pieces and add to the blender together with mint, garlic, dill (have some leftover), vinegar and celery. Blend until smooth and if it's a little thick use the seed to make it thinner.

iii.   Take some salt and the pepper to taste then mix and place it in the refrigerator to chill until the time to serve.

iv.   Dice the remaining cucumber into fine sizes which will be used during serving.

v.   Serve the soup in bowls and use the cucumbers to top and add some chopped dill, celery seeds and some drops of olive oil. You can serve a rye bread on the side with each bowl soup.

PEACH GINGER SMOOTHIE
Nutrition
Servings 4
Calorie 51
Carbohydrate 9g
Protein 2g
Fat 1g
Fiber 2g
Sugar 6g

Ingredients
- 2 yellow peaches, medium sized, pitted and quartered
- 1 tablespoon minced ginger
- 1 orange, peeled
- Orange zest, from orange
- 1 tablespoon grounded flaxseed
- ½ cup milk, unsweetened, cashew, almond or soy
- 2 cups ice cubes

Preparation
To start with, pour all the ingredients in the blender but make sure you use 1 cup of the ice first. Blend them until you can see that the solution has thickened and the smooth solution is achieved, which should be within 1 minute. Add the remaining cup of ice and continue to blend them for a thick smoothie.

You can use extra milk to make the smoothie to the thinness and the desired consistency.

Serve in glasses while still chilled.

SCRAMBLED EGGS WITH CHEDDAR CHEESE
Nutrition
Servings 1
Calories 455
Fat 39g
Carbohydrates 1g
Sugar 1g
Protein 25g

Ingredients
- 2 eggs

- ½ cup cheddar cheese, grated
- 1 tablespoon butter/olive oil
- Salt and pepper to taste
- 2 slice whole grain toasts

Preparation

i. Place a pan on a heater on medium level and add to it the butter.
ii. Beat the eggs in a bowl and whisk with a fork.
iii. Mix the salt and pepper to the egg mixture.
iv. Pour the egg mixture into the frying pan then use the cheese to top a layer. Pull the egg back and forth as the egg mixes with cheese so that to ensure that the egg does not overcook to form the scrabble.
v. When the egg is no longer watery, it is ready to be served on the toasts preferably hot.

https://hurrythefoodup.com/scrambled-eggs-with-cheese/

CHICKPEA SCRAMBLE BREAKFAST

Nutrition

Servings 4
Calories 258
Sugar 1.5g
Fat 10.6g
Carbohydrates 44.6g
Fiber 13.6g
Protein 22.7g

Ingredients

- 15 ounces canned chickpeas, drained
- 2 tablespoon lemon juice
- 2 tablespoon nutritional yeast
- 1 teaspoon garlic powder
- ½ teaspoon turmeric powder
- ¼ teaspoon ground black pepper
- ¼ teaspoon seas salt
- 6 tablespoons hummus

Preparation

i. Take the chickpeas and lemon juice and put in a bowl and mix them thoroughly by mashing with a fork.
ii. Add to the mixture the hummus and the spices then continue mashing so that they are well combined.
iii. Use a medium-high oven for cooking the chickpea in a pan for about 5 minutes while occasionally stirring so that it attains a golden brown appearance. Kindly note that you do not need to add any liquid or cooking oil while doing this.

iv.   The meal is ready to serve for breakfast with some side serves like brown fried mushrooms, avocado, bread, and cherry tomatoes.

v.   If you have some remainder, you can store for up to 5 days in the fridge in a sealed tight container.

https://simpleveganblog.com/easy-chickpea-scramble-10-minutes/

Hormonal Imbalance Recipes

BREAKFAST

DETOXING BEET AND CARROT SALAD

Nutrition

Servings 3

Calories 72

Fats 1.5g

Cholesterol 0mg

Carbohydrates 13.2g

Fiber 3.8g

Sugars 6.9g

Proteins 1.8g

Ingredients

- 1.5 cups carrots, shredded
- 1 cup beets, grated
- 1 medium apple, diced
- 1 cucumber, diced
- 2 tablespoon dried cranberries
- ¼ cup olive oil
- Juice from 1 lemon

Preparation

i.   Take a large bowl and place all the veggies in it then combine them, making sure they are well mixed.

ii.   Whisk the olive and the lemon together to use it for the dressing. Once mixed, pour into the veggies mixture and mix to form an even coating.

iii.   Have the salad chilled by placing it in a fridge for about 20 minutes before serving.

CARROT LEMONADE

Nutrition

Servings 6

Calories 107

Fat 0g

Cholesterol 0g

Carbohydrates 27g

Fiber 3g

Sugar 17g

Protein 1g

Ingredients

- 1 pound carrots, peeled and cut into chucks
- 2 cups water
- 3 cups pineapple juice and unsweetened white grape juice
- ¾ cup lemon juice
- Cold water
- Ice

Preparation

i. Boil the carrots in a medium-sized saucepan before reducing the heat and allowing it to simmer for about 30 minutes or until when they are very tender. Let it cool slightly then transfer the mixture into a blender. Add the pineapple juice and blend while covered until the mixture is smooth.

ii. Transfer into a plastic container then adds the remaining pineapple and lemon juice before mixing. Add some water into the mixture as you desire to make sure that it does not thicken too much when it stands.

iii. Place the solution in the fridge to chill for about 2 to 24 hours.

iv. When ready to drink, serve with ice cubes and lemon wedges.

https://www.bhg.com/recipe/drinks/carrot-lemonade/#nutrition

ROASTED GARLIC PARMESAN CAULIFLOWER

Nutrition

Servings 6

Calories 247

Fat 18g

Cholesterol 48mg

Carbohydrates 14g

Fiber 1g

Sugars 1g

Protein 6g

Ingredients

- ½ cup butter, melted
- 2 garlic cloves, minced
- 1 cup plain breadcrumbs
- ½ cup parmesan cheese, grated
- ¼ teaspoon salt
- ¼ teaspoon black pepper

- 1 cauliflower head, medium size

Preparation

i. Switch on the oven and turn the heat to 400 degrees Fahrenheit then prepare on the side a baking sheet by lining it with a parchment paper.

ii. Pluck the leaves from the cauliflower and cut it into florets preferable of the same size.

iii. Put the melted butter into a bowl then add into it the garlic then stir well.

iv. Take the crumbs, salt, black pepper and the cheese in a different bowl and mix. Take each of the cauliflower and dip into the butter before mixing it with the breadcrumbs. Repeat for all the pieces.

v. When all the cauliflowers are done, place one by one on the earlier prepared baking sheet. Place them into the oven then bake. Preferably for 35 minutes.

vi. When they have turn golden brown, remove from the oven and serve.

https://www.crunchycreamysweet.com/roasted-garlic-parmesan-cauliflower/

PROTEIN PACKED BERRY FROZEN YOGURT

Nutrition

Servings 4

Calorie 124

Carbohydrate 21g

Protein 8g

Fat 1g

Cholesterol 3mg

Fiber 4g

Sugar 14g

Ingredients

- 3 cups frozen strawberries
- 1 cup frozen raspberries
- 1 cup vanilla Greek yoghurt
- 1 scoop of protein vanilla flavor
- 2 tablespoons honey or low calorie sweetener

Preparation

i. Using a food processor bowl, take the frozen berries, the yogurt, protein scoop, and honey.

ii. Blend the mixture until you notice that it is smooth enough. 5 minutes should be enough to attain this.

iii. You can either serve when ready or put into a freezer until you are ready to serve.

iv. If you had kept the yogurt in the freezer, let it to sit for about 5 minutes in the room temperature then serve.

https://healthyfitnessmeals.com/berry-frozen-yogurt/

BACON CHEESEBURGER PIZZA BALLS

Nutrition

Servings 6

Calories 370

Carbohydrates 35g

Fat 17g

Fiber 2g

Sugar 3g

Protein 20g

Ingredients

- 10 refrigerator biscuits
- ½ cup shredded cheddar cheese
- ½ cup browned hamburger pieces
- ¼ cup crispy bacon bits
- Black pepper to taste
- Onion powder
- Egg white, beaten
- Parmesan cheese, grated

Preparation

i. Turn on the oven and adjust the heat to 425 degrees Fahrenheit.

ii. Spread the biscuits dough and then put the mozzarella cheese, cheddar cheese, hamburger pieces, and bacon bits.

iii.   Take the black pepper and onion powders and sprinkle on the top. You can add the cheese as you desire.

iv.   Pick the edges to fold in the toppings and then pinch the top together. Grease the pie pan then place the pizza ball on it.

v.   Place them the folded part on the bottom then use a brush to apply the egg white.

vi.   Take the grated parmesan cheese then use it to sprinkle the top.

vii.   Place them in the heated up oven and bake for 15 minutes so that they are golden brown.

viii.   When ready, take them from the oven and serve with ketchup and pickle slices on the side.

https://www.thegunnysack.com/bacon-cheeseburger-pizza-balls-recipe/

PEANUT BUTTER MOUSSE

Nutrition

Servings 4

Calories 301

Carbohydrates 4g

Fiber 1g

Fats 30g

Proteins 5g

Ingredients

- ½ cup heavy whipping cream
- 4 ounces cream cheese, softened
- ¼ cup natural peanut butter, sugarless
- ¼ cup swerve sweetener, powder
- ½ teaspoon vanilla extract

Preparation

i.   Using a medium-sized bowl, whip the cream until you see it holds stiff peaks then place it aside.

ii.   Take a different same sized bowl and beat the cream cheese together with peanut butter to the point that you achieve a smooth and creamy mix.

iii. Mix the sweetener and vanilla to the peanut butter and add a pinch of salt and continue beating until they have combined and formed a smooth mixture.

iv. In case the mixture is not too smooth, you can add some heavy cream, about 2 tablespoons, and continue beating until it unthickens and is well combined.

v. Take the whipped cream and fold gently until none is remaining. Take the dessert glasses and scoop the mixture into each of them.

vi. You can prepare a low carb chocolate sauce on the side and use it as a drizzled top, but it is optional.

https://alldayidreamaboutfood.com/low-carb-5-minute-peanut-butter-mousse/

LEMON TUNA & YOGURT CRACKER
Nutrition
Serving 1
Calorie 77
Carbohydrate 8g
Protein 10g
Cholesterol 19mg
Fiber 1g
Sugar 1g

Ingredients
- 2 tablespoon tuna, chunk-light
- 2 tablespoons plain Greek yogurt, low-fat
- ¼ teaspoon lemon zest, plus for garnish
- 1 large crisp-bread, whole grain
- 1 teaspoon dill, for garnish

Preparation
i. Take a small bowl and use it to mix the tuna, yogurt together with lemon zest.

ii. Use a spoon to spread the mixture a crisp-bread then use the dill plus the additional zest to garnish them.

iii. Serve the meal for breakfast.

https://www.copymethat.com/r/rPcbZsn/lemon-tuna-yogurt-cracker/

PUMPKIN PORRIDGE
Nutrition
Servings 6
Calorie 192
Carbohydrate 46g

Protein 3g
Fiber 4g
Sugar 12g
Iron 1.7mg

Ingredients

- 1.7kg kabocha /kent pumpkin/butternut squash
- 3 cups water
- ¼ cup sweet rice flour
- 3 tablespoon water
- 3 tablespoon sugar
- ½ teaspoon fine seas salt

Preparation

i. Slice the pumpkin to about 4 sizes of quadrant shapes so that you can be able to remove the seed and strings with a knife or a spoon.

ii. Using a steamer, cook the pumpkins to the point that they are tender and soft. Place them on the side and cut the skin off so that you remain with the flesh alone. The pumpkin can now be further cut into smaller chunks.

iii. Place the sliced pumpkins into a blender with water, sugar and the salt then blend to the point that they are pureed. Transfer the liquid into a saucepan where you will cook to boiling point for about 10 mines. Make sure you stir while they cook in the order they do not burn.

iv. Take the rice flour and some water about 3 tablespoons into a bowl and mix them to combine. Transfer into a larger saucepan with pumpkin porridge to stir so that there will be no lumps. Place the porridge over low heat to simmer to about 3 minutes.

v. If you love some rice cake balls, you can garnish the porridge with them when serving.

https://mykoreankitchen.com/pumpkin-porridge-hobakjuk/

GRAIN-FREE CEREALS WITH PEARS

Nutrition

Servings 4
Calorie 1018
Carbohydrate 150g
Protein 5g
Fat 48g
Sugar 29g
Sodium 106mg

Ingredients

- 900 grams apples, peeled and sliced

- ¼ cup maple syrup
- 1 teaspoon vanilla extract
- ½ cup unsalted butter
- 1 ¼ cups regular rolled oats
- 1/3 cup whole wheat flour
- ½ cup packed light brown sugar
- 1 teaspoon ground cinnamon
- Pinch salt

Preparation

i. Place the oven's knob to position 350 degrees Fahrenheit. Transfer the sliced apple into a large bowl and add maple syrup into the bowl then stir it well while adding vanilla to coat the apple.

ii. Using a saucepan to melt butter on medium-high heat so that it turns brown and the foam subsides then set it aside.

iii. Place the oat, flour, sugar, the cinnamon, and salt into a large bowl and mix thoroughly. Continue blending with browned butter. Take the mixture and spread them over the apples then bake them for about 45 minutes. When done, the apple should be natural to slide when a knife is inserted.

iv. Let the crisp cool down for roughly 15 minutes before you serve.

https://www.lifestylefood.com.au/recipes/25187/warm-apple-crisp

LUNCH

BLACK BEAN TEMPEH NACHOS WITH CASHEW CHEESE

Nutrition
Servings 4
Calorie 772
Carbohydrate 82g
Protein 27g
Fat 34g
Fiber 18g
Sugar 4g

Ingredients
- 14 ounces tortilla chips, packed
- 14 ounces black beans, canned
- 8 ounces tempeh, very small dices
- ½ cup red onion, diced
- 1 hot chili pepper, sliced thinly
- 1 Roma tomato, diced small
- 2 tablespoons hempseed, raw shelled
- 1 avocado, sliced
- 1 tablespoon lime juice
  For Cashew Nacho Cheese
- ¾ raw cashews, soaked overnight
- ½ cup water
- 1 tablespoon nutritional yeast
- 2 teaspoons tapioca starch
- ½ teaspoon garlic powder
- ½ teaspoon onion powder
- 2 teaspoon lemon juice, fresh lemon

Preparation
Cashew Cheese

i. Take the overnight soaked cashews and drain the water. Add the ingredients for preparing the cashew cheese together into a blender and blend until you attain a smooth solution.

ii. Transfer the blended solution into a pan and cook, ensuring that the heat is at its medium level.

iii. The cooking should continue to the point that you realize that the sauce has thickened before removing from the heat. That should take about 5 minutes.

Nacho Assembly

i. Take the chips and lay them on a platter. From the ingredients, use the beans, diced tomatoes, pepper and tempeh to sprinkle over the chips.
ii. Use the cashew cream to dot before sprinkling the red onions, pepper, and hempseed over the meal.
iii. Pick the avocado and dredge in lime juice before topping the nachos.
iv. Serve and enjoy for lunch.

https://veganinthefreezer.com/vegan-nachos/

MUSHROOM BURGER
Nutrition
Servings 6
Calorie 255
Carbohydrate 22.5g
Protein 11.4g
Fat 14.2g
Cholesterol 67mg
Fiber 3.1g
Sugar 4g

Ingredients
- 2 tablespoons olive oil
- 3 packages fresh mushrooms, sliced
- ½ onion, finely chopped
- 4 garlic cloves, minced
- 1 teaspoon salt
- ½ teaspoon black pepper
- ½ teaspoon dried oregano
- 2/3 cup rolled oats
- ¾ cup bread crumbs, dried
- 2 eggs, beaten
- ½ cup freshly shredded Parmigiano-Reggiano cheese
- 2 tablespoons olive oil

Preparation
i. Place a large skillet over a medium heated cooker and add 2 tablespoons of olive oil. Tip into the oil mushrooms, onions, and garlic and use salt and pepper to season.
ii. Cook the mushroom while frequently stirring until you see that the mushroom has lost it juice. This should take about 10 minutes before transferring to the chopping board where you chop the mushrooms to small chunks using a kitchen knife.

iii.   Take a large bowl and pour the mushrooms there and then mic with oats and breadcrumbs. Taste whether the pepper and salt are enough and if not add some to your requirement.

iv.   The cheese and the beaten eggs are ready to be added to the mixture. Stir then allow the mixture to rest for about 15 minutes which helps the crumbs to soak any excess liquid. For later cooking, the combination can be stored in the refrigerator.

v.   Moist your hands with vegetable oil and then scoop about ¼ cup of the mixture and use to make burgers. Repeat until the mixture is entirely done.

vi.   Using some olive oil poured in the skillet, place it over the heat on medium level heat and fry the burgers until you notice that they are turning brown and well cooked. The preparation takes between 5 to 6 minutes.

vii.   Slice the bread roll and serve the mushrooms with some mayonnaise, sliced tomatoes, lettuce or vegetable of your choice just like while serving any other burger.

https://www.allrecipes.com/recipe/233999/mushroom-veggie-burger/

SPANISH PUMPKIN AND CHICKPEA STEW

Nutrition

Servings 2
Calorie 566
Carbohydrate 94.5g
Protein 24.1g
Fat 13.2g
Fiber 21.9g
Sugar 17.2g

Ingredients

- 3 cups water
- 2 cloves of garlic
- ½ onion, chopped
- ¼ green bell pepper, chopped
- ¼ red bell pepper, chopped
- ½ tomato, chopped
- 2 tablespoons tomato paste
- 1 chopped medium potato
- 2 cups chopped raw pumpkin
- 2 teaspoon sweet paprika
- ½ teaspoon ground ginger
- 1 tablespoon extra-virgin olive oil
- 15 ounces cooked/canned chickpeas
- Fresh parsley for garnish

Preparation

i. Place a large pot with water over a cooker and boil. Add the garlic, onion, the peppers, tomato, and tomato paste and cook them over medium-high heat for 5 minutes.

ii. Pour the mixture in a blender and process until the solution is smooth then pour it back into the pot.

iii. Put the potatoes inside and cook for 10 minutes over medium-high heat.

iv. The pumpkins can now be added into the pot and then cooked for about 15 to 20 minutes which will depend on the type of pumpkin you are using.

v. Take the paprika ginger and the oil and add to the soup and stir well,

vi. Add to the solution the chickpeas and cook them for 5 minutes extra.

vii. The meal should be ready to serve and ensure to use the parsley to garnish each soup bowl.

https://simpleveganblog.com/spanish-pumpkin-and-chickpea-stew/

MUSTARDY BEETROOT & LENTIL SALAD

Nutrition

Servings
Calorie 156
Carbohydrate 21g
Protein 10g
Fat 4g
Fiber 6g
Sugar 6g
Salt 0.3g

Ingredients

- 500g packed pre-cooked lentils
- 1 tablespoon wholegrain mustard
- 1 ½ tablespoon extra-virgin olive oil
- 300g pack cooked beetroot, sliced
- Large handful tarragon, roughly chopped

Preparation

i. Follow the instruction on the packets on how to prepare the precooked lentils, drain well, and leave them to cool down.

ii. On the side, take the mustard and combine with oil and do some seasoning in the preparing of the dressing.

iii. Transfer the lentils into a bowl, put the dressing and then mix them well. Add into the mixture the beetroot, tarragon, and some additional seasoning and stir them together.

iv. Serve in a plate and enjoy.

https://www.bbcgoodfood.com/recipes/mustardy-beetroot-lentil-salad

KALE & QUINOA PATTIES

Nutrition

Servings 4

Calorie 564

Carbohydrate 43g

Protein 21g

Fat 33g

Fiber 3g

Sugar 9g

Ingredients

- 140g quinoa
- 500g hot vegetable stock
- 100g kale, stalks removed, leaves roughly chopped
- 3 tablespoon olive oil
- 1 small onion, finely chopped
- 2 garlic cloves, crushed
- 75g fresh white breadcrumbs
- 2 medium eggs, beaten
- 50g sundried tomatoes, roughly chopped
- 100g goat's cheese
- Green salad, to serve
    For Pesto
- ½ small pack basil, leaves only
- ½ small pack parsley, leaves only
- 2 garlic cloves, crushed
- 50g pine nuts, toasted
- 50g parmesan, grated
- 150g olive oil
- Lemon juice, 1 lemon

Preparation

i. Pick a saucepan and place the quinoa in it then add the hot stock and simmer for about 18 to 20 minutes. Ensure that you do not heat too much so that you can cook until the grains fluff up and there is no more liquid left. Place aside from the heat and allow it to cool down.

ii. Boil on the side water in a large saucepan and add the kales then allow them to simmer for 6 to 8 minutes so that they are well cooked. Drain dry the kales including by even squeezing the water from them.

iii. Take a frying pan and put in on medium-high heated cooker and add 1 tablespoon of oil before adding onions to cook for 2 to 3 minutes until they change to translucent. Put the garlic to the same pan and good together with the onions for another 1 minute. Pick the earlier prepared quinoa, kales, onions, breadcrumbs, garlic, egg, and sundried tomatoes. Use the seasoning available and mix them to combine and set it aside.

iv. On the side, you can prepare the pesto with basil, parsley, pine, garlic, and parmesan in a food processor. Beat them together as you slowly pour in the oil so that you achieve a thick pesto. Also, squeeze the lemon juice to the mixture before setting it aside.

v. The next step will be to prepare the patties so place a shallow pan on the heater where you will then add 2 tablespoons of olive oil. Use your hands to make the patties into probably 8 rounds then use the pan to fry them each side of them for 4 to 5 minutes so that they are crispy and golden brown.

vi. Prepare the grill and heat it then use the goat cheese on each patty which you will later place on the grill to brown them more and the cheese to melt. The process does not take too long, so keep watch of the patties.

vii. They should be ready, and you can use pesto and green leaves to top the patties while serving if that is your preference.

https://www.bbcgoodfood.com/recipes/kale-quinoa-patties

HERBED CHICKEN MEATBALL WITH ZOODLES & PESTO
Nutrition
Servings 4
Calorie 470
Carbohydrate 24g
Protein 30g
Fat 5g
Cholesterol 144mg
Fiber 6.5g
Sugar 13g

Ingredients
Meatballs
- 4 ounces Cremini mushrooms, halved
- ½ cup roughly chopped sweet onion
- 2 cloves garlic, roughly chopped
- 1 ½ teaspoons avocado oil
- 1 pound ground chicken
- 1 large egg
- 2 tablespoon unsalted Italian seasoning
- 1 tablespoon ground flaxseed

- 1 tablespoon nutritional yeast
- ½ teaspoon each seas salt and ground black pepper
- 3 cups marinara sauce
  Pesto
- 1 cup fresh basil
- ¼ cup raw unsalted walnuts
- 1 tablespoon nutritional yeast
- 1 tablespoon lemon zest
- 1 tablespoon fresh lemon juice
- 1 clove garlic
- ¼ teaspoon ground black pepper
- 1 tablespoon avocado oil
  Zoodles
- 2 tablespoon avocado oil
- 4 zucchini, done with spiralizer
- Seas salt and ground pepper to taste

Preparation

i. First prepare the meatballs where you begin with making a mixture of mushrooms, onions, and garlic through blending them until they are well minced. Transfer into a moderate size skillet and cook over medium-high heat with oil. The cooking should take at least 4 minutes before transferring to a bowl to cool. Clean the food processor.

ii. Using a parchment, line a baking sheet and set aside. Take the bowl with the mushroom mixture and add the chicken, eggs, seasoning, flaxseed, yeast, salt and black pepper. Combine with your hands in order to do it thoroughly.

iii. By now the mixture should be able to form meatballs when scooped so scoop into the baking sheet you prepared earlier. Place into the cooker and bake for 20 minutes so that they are well cooked.

iv. Take the ingredients for the pesto by putting them into a food processor apart from the oil. Blend them well until they are finely chopped before adding the oil and blending again for another 30 seconds.

v. For the zoodles, pour half of the oil into a none-sticky skillet on medium-high heat and heat then add half of the zucchini with salt and pepper and sauté for 3 to 4 minutes while stirring. Cook the remaining ones the same way as a different potion with the remained oil.

vi. Serve the pesto into the plate, the zoodles and then the meatballs on the top.

https://www.cleaneatingmag.com/recipes/herbed-chicken-meatball-marinara-zoodles-pesto-recipe

BEEF STIR-FRY WITH VEGETABLES
Nutrition

Servings 4
Calories: 277
Carbs: 11g
Protein 32g
Fat 10g
Fiber 1g
Sugar 6g
Serving

Ingredients

- 1 tablespoon vegetable oil, divided
- 1 red bell pepper, sliced into strips
- 1 green bell pepper, sliced into strips
- 1 ¼ pounds flank steak, sliced thinly
- 2 teaspoon minced garlic
- 1 teaspoon minced ginger
- Salt and pepper to taste
- ¼ cup soy sauce
- ¼ cup of water
- 1 ½ tablespoons sugar
- 1 ½ tablespoons cornstarch

Preparation

i. Place a large pan on a medium heated cooker and pour 1 teaspoon of vegetable oil.
ii. Cook the green and red peppers so that to attain the desired tenderness then place them on a plate.
iii. Use the same pan to add the remaining oil then take the steak while seasoned with pepper and salt. Make sure that the heat has been adjusted to high.
iv. Cook the stead on the pan for more than 5 minutes or until you achieve a light brownish look.
v. Add to the steak the ginger and garlic and mix then continue cooking for about 30 seconds.
vi. Take the cooked peppers and add them back to the pan with the steak.
vii. Put the remaining ingredients in a small bowl then whisk then thoroughly to form a sauce.
viii. Use the sauce over the steak mixture and bring the meal to simmer. Allow the meal to cook for another 2 to 3 minutes so that you have the sauce thicker.
ix. You can best serve it with brown rice on the side.

https://www.dinneratthezoo.com/pepper-steak-stir-fry/

PUMPKIN SEED CRUSTED CHICKEN SALAD

Nutrition

Servings 2
Calories 240

Fat 10.8g
Carbohydrates 19g
Fiber 3.7g
Sugars 3g
Protein 17.7g

Ingredients
Main
- 8 chicken tenders
- 1/3 cup breadcrumbs
- 1/3 cup pumpkin seeds, cut in smaller pieces
- 1 egg
- Salt and pepper to taste
- 3 tablespoons frying oil
- 2 handfuls leaf lettuce
- 8 small tomatoes
- ½ greenhouse cucumber
- 1 small red onion

For Dressing
- 2 tablespoons pumpkin seed oil
- 1 tablespoon apple cider vinegar
- 1 teaspoon Dijon mustard
- 1 teaspoon honey
- Salt and pepper to taste

Preparation
i.   Use the salt and pepper to season the chicken tenders after slicing it into equal pieces. Take the eggs and beat with a fork on the side then on another plate, put pumpkin seeds and the breadcrumbs and mix them thoroughly.

ii. Take the chicken pieces and place each in the beaten eggs then coat them with the breadcrumbs mixture. Try to coat the chicken with bread as much as possible so that the breadcrumbs are used up.

iii. Place a frying pan on a highly heated cooker and add the frying oil then cook the chicken making sure that you turn both sides and they attain a golden look. Line a plate with paper towels and transfer the chicken there.

iv. Take the dressing ingredients and put in a small jar then add pepper and salt to taste and shake them thoroughly.

v.   Wash the lettuce clean and spread them on plates then top them with the chicken pieces. Slice the tomatoes into half, cut the cucumber into small pieces and the onions too then add to the toppings.

vi. Take the sauce and pour over the meal and serve it for lunch or dinner.

FRITTATA WITH VEGETABLES

Nutrition

Servings 6

Calories 177

Fat 12g

Cholesterol 213mg

Carbohydrates 10g

Sugars 3g

Fiber 2g

Protein 8g

Ingredients

- ½ cup of chopped onions
- ½ cup of chopped green pepper
- ½ cup of chopped red pepper
- 1 garlic clove, minced
- 3 tablespoons olive oil, divided
- 2 medium red potatoes, cooked and cubed
- 1 small zucchini, cubed
- 6 large eggs
- ½ teaspoon salt
- Pinch of pepper

Preparation

i. Take an ovenproof skillet and put in it the prepared onions, peppers plus garlic and sauté over a preheated broiler in 2 tablespoons of the oil so that they are tender enough. Serve the veggies off the skillet and place on the side.

ii. Cook in the same skillet the potatoes with the remaining oil until they are brownish then add to it the vegetables and zucchini. Let the food cook for about 4 minutes.

iii. Beat the eggs in a bowl, making sure you mix them with salt and pepper then pour to the cooking vegetables. Place the cover on the skillet and allow them to cook for about 8 minutes so as the eggs are nearly set.

iv. Let the meal rest for about 2 minutes so that the egg can set well on the top then serve in cut wedges just like a pizza.

LEMON HERB SALMON & VEGGIES

Nutrition

Servings 4

Calories 326

Fat 20g
Carbs 8g
Fiber 2g
Sugar 3g
Protein 27g

Ingredients

- 1 tablespoon garlic, minced
- 1 tablespoon dried rosemary
- 1 tablespoon dried oregano
- 1 tablespoon dried basil
- 1 tablespoon olive oil
- 1 tablespoon lemon juice
- 4 fillets salmon
- 1 large zucchini, chopped
- 75 grams of mushroom, sliced
- 1 yellow bell pepper, sliced
- 470 grams of cherry tomatoes, halved
- Olive oil
- Salt and pepper to taste

Preparation

i.   Take the oven heat up to 200 degrees Celsius as you prepare the other ingredients.

ii. In a bowl, mix well the herbs, garlic, lemon juice, olive oil, salt, and pepper.

iii. Using baking sheet lined with parchment paper, place the salmon on one half and cover it with at least 1/3 of the herb mixture then flip and cover it with the remaining mixture.

iv. Put the remaining vegetables on the remaining half and mix them then spread. Drizzle the olive oil, remaining salt and pepper to the meal.

v.   Place them in the baker and cook for 30 minutes which will make the tomatoes to burst and the salmon will be easy to flake.

vi. Remove from the oven and allow it to rest before serving for lunch or dinner.

https://tasty.co/recipe/one-pan-lemon-herb-salmon-veggies

WARM LENTIL AND TOMATO SALAD

Nutrition

Servings 2
Calories 190
Fat 5g
Carbohydrates 25g
Sugars 5g
Fiber 6g
Protein 11g

Ingredients

- 120grams of brown lentils
- 10 sun dried tomatoes
- 3 sprigs fresh parsley
- 1 tablespoon balsamic vinegar
- 1 tablespoon lemon juice
- 1 tablespoon maple syrup
- 2 teaspoon olive oil, divided
- ¼ teaspoon Dijon mustard
- 14 ounces can chickpeas
- 1 teaspoon chili powder
- 1 pinch ground cumin
- ¼ teaspoon ground turmeric
- 1 pinch sea salt

Preparation

i. Power the oven and preheat to 200 degrees Celsius. Drain chickpeas dry with a kitchen paper to male them moisture free for roasting.

ii. Put the chickpeas in the bowl and add olive oil then mix well and add spices so that they are evenly coated. Take a parchment paper and lay it on a baking sheet and put in the oven then bake for 20 minutes. Allow them to cool down well so that they can become crispier.

iii. Cook the lentils on the side with a saucepan by boiling them for 25 to 30 minutes until they are well done. Take the balsamic vinegar, lemon juice, maple, olive, and mustard in a separate bowl and whisk them thoroughly together.

iv. Remove the lentils to drain water and then place them back in the saucepan then put the dressing. Allow them to rest together for 5 to 10 minutes for proper absorption. Slice the tomatoes then chop the parsley before mixing them with the lentils.

v. The meal is ready to be served with quinoas and avocado slices on the side.

http://laurencariscooks.com/warm-lentil-tomato-salad/

CRANBERRY APPLE PECAN QUINOA SALAD

Nutrition

Servings 6
Calories 372
Fat 23.4g
Carbohydrates 35.7g
Fiber 5.1g
Protein 8.3g
Sugars 12g

Ingredients

- 1 ½ cups of chicken broth
- 1 cup quinoa, rinsed
- 3 tablespoons olive oil
- 1 ½ tablespoons Dijon mustard
- 1 teaspoon maple syrup
- ¼ teaspoon ground cinnamon
- Salt and black pepper grounded to taste
- 1 large crisp apple, chopped
- 1 cup pecan pieces
- ½ cup dried cranberries
- ½ cup grated parmesan cheese

Preparation

i. Place the chicken broth and quinoa in a saucepan and stir fry until you bring to boiling then low the heat. Cover the saucepan and let the meal cook for another 10 minutes so that all the broth has been absorbed. Transfer the pan from the heat and fluff the food with a fork.

ii. Put the olive, Dijon, maple syrup and cinnamon in a bowl then whisk them together. Use the salt and black pepper to season.

iii. Slice the apple into small pieces and add together with pecan, cranberries plus parmesan cheese to the mixture and stir well. Cover the saucepan again for 5 to 10 minutes and allow the mixture to steam for the sauce to warm up and the apples become softer.

iv. Mixed salad should be ready to serve in 6 portions.

https://www.allrecipes.com/recipe/234447/cranberry-apple-pecan-quinoa-salad/

CREAMY CHICKEN LIVER AND ZOODLES

Nutrition

Servings 2
Calories 590
Fat 48g

Cholesterol 535mg
Carbohydrates 16g
Fiber 4g
Sugars 5g
Protein 25g

Ingredients

- 1 large onion, sliced
- 2 garlic cloves, crushed
- 250grams of chicken liver
- 2 tablespoons of coconut oil
- ½ cup double cream, divided
- ½ teaspoon paprika
- ¼ teaspoon oregano
- Salt and pepper to taste
- 1 large zucchini
- ¼ tablespoon of butter

Preparation

i. Make sure that the livers are sinew and fat-free before slicing them into small portions, then wash them well before drying them with a kitchen paper.

ii. Heat the coconut oil in the skillet then add onions then cook until they become tender before adding the garlic and the liver.

iii. Cook the liver while stirring for about 6 minutes then season with paprika, marjoram, salt and pepper as you stir. Once they are well mixed, cover the skillet and allow the cooking to go on for about 5 minutes. Add some water if the need arises to avoid sticking on the skillet and make sure the liver does not overcook.

iv. Add the cream and stir to boil before removing the skillet off the heater.

v. On the side, prepare the zucchini into zoodles with a Spiralizer. Cook them in another skillet for about 2 minutes with some butter.

vi. Serve the zoodles on a plate then the creamy liver on top and enjoy for lunch or dinner.

http://myzucchinirecipes.com/creamy-liver-and-onions-with-zoodles/

VEGAN TURMERIC QUINOA POWER BOWLS

Nutrition

Servings 4
Calories 385
Sugar 3g
Fat 18g
Carbohydrates 53g
Protein 15g
Cholesterol 0g

Ingredients
- 7 small yellow potatoes
- 15 ounces of canned chickpeas
- 2 teaspoon turmeric, divided
- 1 teaspoon paprika
- 1 tablespoon coconut oil
- ¼ cup quinoa
- Salt and pepper to taste
- 2 kale leaves
- ½ teaspoon olive oil
- 1 avocado

Preparation
i. Power on the oven and adjust the temperature up to 350 Fahrenheit in advance.
ii. As the oven heats, slice on the side the potatoes preferably into small strips then take a baking sheet and lay them on one half of it. Spray the coconut oil, sprinkle a tablespoon of turmeric. Add the salt and/or pepper to taste.
iii. Place in the oven and roast for about five minutes.
iv. Take the chickpeas and drain well before putting them in a mixing bowl. Take paprika and add to the bowl then mix them to coat evenly. Remove the baking sheet from the oven and spread the chickpeas on the remaining half of the baking sheet.
v. Place them back to the oven and bake for another 25 minutes so that the chickpeas cook well and the potatoes soften.
vi. Put the quinoa in a pan and cook with a ½ cup of water then add the remaining turmeric then salt and pepper to taste and mix well before letting it cool down.
vii. Take the kales and wash them thoroughly and use the olive oil to apply on the leaves before spreading on the bowl.
viii. Slice the avocado into pieces and put in the bowl then serve the quinoa, chickpeas and roasted potatoes on the bowl for breakfast.

https://www.jaroflemons.com/vegan-turmeric-quinoa-power-bowls/

SALMON PASTA SALAD

Nutrition

Servings 4

Calories 332

Fats 18g

Cholesterol 23mg

Carbohydrates 27g

Fiber 3g

Sugars 4g

Protein 16g

Ingredients

- 8 ounces spiral pasta, cooked and drained
- 2 cups salmon chunks, fully cooked
- 1 ½ cherry tomatoes, quartered
- 1 medium size cucumber, quartered and sliced
- 1 small red onion, sliced
- ½ cup canola oil
- 1/3 cup lemon juice
- 1 ½ teaspoons dill weed
- 1 garlic clove, minced
- ¾ teaspoon salt
- ¼ teaspoon pepper
- 1 head lettuce, torn

Preparation

i. Mix first the pasta, salmon, tomatoes, cucumber, and onions in a bowl.

ii. On the side, take the lemon, dill weed, garlic, salt, and pepper and mix them well to form a solution for dressing.

iii. Mix both the mixture and the dressing and then cover before placing it in the fridge to chill for about 20 minutes.

iv. Serve while chilled with some lettuce laid over the plate.

https://www.tasteofhome.com/recipes/salmon-pasta-salad/

CAULIFLOWER FRIED RICE

Nutrition

Servings 4

Calories 273

Fat 17g

Carbohydrates 22g

Sugar 8g

Fiber 7g

Protein 12g

Cholesterol 93mg

Ingredients

- Vegetable oil
- 2 large eggs, beaten
- Salt to taste
- 1 cup chopped scallions, green parts and light parts separate
- 3 garlic cloves, minced
- 1 tablespoon fresh ginger, finely chopped
- 2 pounds cauliflower
- 5 tablespoons soy sauce, gluten free
- ¼ teaspoon red pepper flakes
- 1 teaspoon sugar
- 1 cup frozen peas and carrots
- 1 teaspoon rice vinegar
- 1 teaspoon Asian sesame oil
- ¼ cup chopped cashews, peanuts

Preparation

i. Use a food processor fit with grating disk to prepare the cauliflower. Use this process when using fresh cauliflower.

ii. Using a large and yet nonstick skillet, place it on medium heat then add into it 2 teaspoons of the vegetable oil. Put the beaten eggs plus a pinch of salt and cook the egg as scrambled. Serve the scramble on a small plate then place it aside.

iii. Clean the pan and place it back in the heater and add 3 tablespoons of veg oil. To it put garlic, scallions, ginger and cook for 3 to 4 minutes while stirring to achieve soft and brown mix.

iv.   Take the cauliflower while grated, the soy sauce, red pepper, sugar and ¼ teaspoon of salt. Cook for about 3 minutes while stirring.

v.   Add into the mixture the peas and carrots then cook for a few minutes until the cauliflowers are a bit crispy yet tender and the veggies have warmed up.

vi.   Finally add the remaining ingredients like vinegar, sesame, dark green scallions, nuts, and eggs and stir them well. Taste to confirm the seasoning is well before serving for lunch.

https://www.onceuponachef.com/recipes/cauliflower-fried-rice.html

CAULIFLOWER PIZZA CRUST

Servings 4

Calories 74

Fat 4g

Carbohydrates 4g

Fiber 2g

Protein 6g

Ingredients

- 2 pounds cauliflower florets, riced
- 1 egg, beaten
- 1/3 cup soft goat cheese
- 1 teaspoon dried oregano
- Salt to taste

Preparation

i.   Make sure you prepare a fresh or frozen cauliflower into riced one.

ii.   Boil the riced cauliflower until its tender then drains the water and transfer to a dishtowel where you will squeeze to drain the extra liquid. You should have a dry and nice pizza crust.

iii.   Transfer the rice into a larger bowl where you will add egg, cheese, and spices and mix well with your hands. The texture may not be like pizza dough, but it is nothing to worry since they will hold well. Just ensure you mix them thoroughly.

iv. Lay the dough on a baking sheet which has been laid well with a parchment paper. Ensure that the mixture is thick but not very thick. About ½ an inch is okay, and the edges can be left a bit thicker than the rest of the spread dough.

v. Place the dough in an already preheated oven at about 400 degrees Fahrenheit and let it cook for about 30 to 35 minutes. When it is golden and tough, then it is ready. Flip the crust and cook again for about 10 to 15 minutes so that it nicely dry's.

vi. Add the pizza topping with your preferred cheese and return in the oven to cook for5 to 10 minutes. The cheese will be a bit bubbly before you remove from the oven.

vii. Remove from the oven and slice into equal slices and serve to four people.

https://detoxinista.com/the-secret-to-perfect-cauliflower-pizza-crust/

RHUBARB CRUMBLE

Nutrition

Servings 4

Calories 440

Fats 18g

Carbohydrates 68g

Sugar 42g

Fiber 3g

Protein 4g

Ingredients

- 500 grams rhubarb, chopped into chunks
- 100 grams golden caster sugar
- 3 tablespoon port
- 140 grams self-rising flour
- 85 grams butter, chilled
- 50 grams light brown muscovado sugar
- 50g chopped walnuts

Preparation

i. Put together the rhubarbs, caster sugar and the port in a saucepan on a low heated cooker and allow them to simmer for about 15 minutes. They should cook until the rhubarb is soft but must maintain its shape at the end then pour it in a medium-sized baking dish

ii. Switch on the oven and let it heat up to 200oC. On the side be preparing the toppings which involve the rubbing of the flour and the chilled butter using your fingers until you attain a soft but crumbled topping.

iii. Take the muscovado sugar and walnuts then add to the mixture and continue mixing with your hands. By now the topping is ready so scatter it over rhubarb then place it in the oven to cook for 30 minutes until when it is golden brown color on top then remove from the oven.

iv. Serve the crumble while still hot and so enjoy it for your lunch or dinner.

https://www.bbcgoodfood.com/recipes/420616/rhubarb-crumble

CRUSTY PARMESAN HERB ZUCCHINI

Nutrition

Serves 4

Calories 255

Carbohydrates 18g

Protein 10g

Fat 16g

Fat 9g

Cholesterol 41mg

Fiber 3g

Sugar 8g

Ingredients

- 4 large zucchini, halved lengthwise
- 2/3 cup panko breadcrumbs
- ½ cup fresh grated parmesan cheese

- ¼ cup finely chopped parsley
- 4 cloves garlic, minced
- ¼ cup melted butter
- Salt and pepper to taste

Preparation

i. Take a baking tray and spray with non-stick oil and set it aside. At the same time, power the oven and heat it in advance to 400 degrees Fahrenheit.

ii. Pick the zucchini and place them one by one on the sheet making sure that the cut side faces up. Put that aside.

iii. Select the breadcrumbs, cheese, parsley, and garlic and mix them thoroughly together in a small bowl.

iv. Take the melted butter and pour to the mixture then add salt and pepper to taste. Take the ingredients, put together, and mix so that the breadcrumbs absorb the butter entirely.

v. Use the spoon to spread the mixture over every zucchini so that they are evenly covered. Use an oil spray to spray some oil on the top.

vi. Place them into the oven and cook or about 20 minutes which should make the crust turn golden brown and the zucchini will be well cooked.

vii. Reduce the heat into medium-high and allow the meal to broil for another 5 minutes before turning the oven off.

viii. Use the parsley to garnish. The zucchinis can be served on the side as an accompaniment during any main meal.

https://cafedelites.com/parmesan-crusted-zucchini/

Sugar 6g

Ingredients

- 1 ¼ pounds ocean perch fillets
- 2 cups frozen peas, thawed
- 1 cup fresh button mushrooms, halved
- ¼ cup grape tomatoes
- 1 small onion, thinly cut in wedges
- 4 teaspoons olive oil, divided

- ¼ teaspoon black pepper, grounded, divided
- 2 teaspoons snipped dill, fresh

Preparation

i.   Use a paper towel to fry up the fish after rinsing it with water. Slice the fillets to fit four servings.

ii. Switch on the oven, turn the knob to heat it at 425 degrees Fahrenheit. Use a cooking spray to sprig a light coat over a baking sheet.

iii. Use a medium-sized bowl to combine the peas with mushrooms, onions, and tomatoes. Take 3 teaspoons of oil and drizzle over the ingredients then sprinkle with about a 1/8 of salt and pepper; coat by tossing them together.

iv. Take the prepared pan and place the vegetables on one side and place them in the oven to cook for 10 minutes.

v.   Remove the pan and arrange the fillets on the remaining section then use the remaining oil on them using a brush and sprinkle the salt and pepper too. Stir the vegetables before roasting again for 12 minutes. Once the fish flakes and the veggies are tender, then you can have the meal removed from the oven.

vi. Serve the meals in portions and after sprinkling the dill.

http://www.eatingwell.com/recipe/264334/oven-roasted-fish-with-peas-and-tomatoes/

HALIBUT WITH CREAMED SPINACH

Nutrition

Servings 2

Calorie 788

Carbohydrate 21g

Protein 43g

Fat 61g

Cholesterol 207mg

Fiber 5g

Sugar 9g

Ingredients

For Seared Halibut

- 12 ounces halibut fillets, 2 six ounces each
- Sea salt to taste
- Black pepper to taste
- 1 ounce vegetable oil

For Creamed Spinach

- 2 tablespoons butter
- 1 tablespoon olive oil
- 1 Vidalia onion, minced
- 1 clove garlic, minced
- 12 ounces baby spinach, stems removed
- ¼ teaspoon ground nutmeg
- ½ cup heavy cream
- ¼ cup Romano cheese, grated

Preparation

i. Take the sea salt and the pepper and apply on the fillets to season each side before undertaking the process of searing.

ii. Place a large steel pan on a large heated cooker and then pour oil enough to coat the better section of the pan and then let the oil heat to the point it starts shimmering.

iii. Place the fillets on the oil and lightly press with a spatula so that there is contact with the bottom of the pan. This should be done every 30 seconds of cooking until 3 minutes are over.

iv. Reduce the heat lower to medium level and then turn the other side of the fish. The cooking should be 2 to 4 minutes repeating the process as above. Make sure that you do not overcook the fillets.

v. In preparing the spinach, place a sauté pan on the heat at a medium-high level, melt the butter and add olive.

vi. Take the onions and mix with garlic then cook them for about 2 minutes so that they become soft.

vii. Put the spinach into the ingredients cooking and sauté until they have wilted. At this level, they are ready to be flavored with salt, pepper, nutmeg, cheese, and the cream. Mix them well when the heat is reduced to medium level.

viii. The cooking should continue until the liquid reduces and the sauce thickens for about 5 to 6 minutes.

ix. Turn off the heat and serve the spinach while still hot and place the halibut fillets on top.

https://www.askchefdennis.com/pan-seared-halibut/

KIDNEY BEAN BURRITO BOWL
Nutrition
Servings 8
Calorie 393
Carbohydrate 59g
Protein 14g
Fat 12g
Cholesterol 17mg
Fiber 7g
Sugar 6g

Ingredients
- 2 tablespoons canola oil
- 1 cup chopped red onions, divided
- 2 teaspoons minced garlic
- 2 cups brown rice, uncooked
- 2 cans Hunts Tomato sauce, no salt added
- 3 ½ cups water
- 4 teaspoons ground Chile pepper
- 1 ¼ teaspoons ground cumin, divided
- 1 can black beans, drained and rinsed
- 1 can garbanzo beans, drained and rinsed

- 1 can diced tomatoes and green chilies, drained
- ½ cup sweet kernel corn, cooked and cooled
- ¼ cup chopped fresh cilantro
- 1 tablespoon lime juice
- ½ teaspoon hot pepper sauce
- ½ teaspoon kosher salt
- 1 ½ cups shredded reduced fat Mexican cheese blend
- 2 cups shredded romaine lettuce
- ½ cup reduced fat sour cream

Preparation

i. Place a medium-sized saucepan and place it over the heat that is medium-level then add the oil until hot. Pour about 2/3 cup of the onions into the oil and the garlic then cook for 5 minutes until they are tender – stir while cooking them. Add the rice and cook for 2 minutes while stirring.

ii. Pour tomato sauce, water, grounded Chile and cumin (1 teaspoon) into the pan and let them come to boiling. Lower the level of the heat and cover to allow about 45 minutes simmering the liquid in the food is absorbed.

iii. While the rice cooks, take a large bowl and in it mix the beans, tomatoes, corn, remained onions, cilantro, lime juice, hot sauce, and the balance cumin and mix well before setting it aside.

iv. The rice should be ready so stir in it some salt to taste and then divide it into portions of the servings on in a large dish. Use the cheese, lettuce, and the beans mixture you prepared as toppings.

v. The meal can be served immediately and use the sour cream as the final topping of each serving.

https://www.readyseteat.com/recipes-Bean-Burrito-Bowl-4275

GRILLED AVOCADO, CAULIFLOWER AND SWEET POTATO

Nutrition
Servings 4
Calorie 467
Carbohydrate 46.2g
Protein 10.9g
Fat 26g
Fiber 15.7g
Sugar 8.2g

Ingredients

Main Ingredients
- 2 medium sweet potatoes, 600 grams

- Salt
- 2 large zucchinis
- 4 cups cauliflower, cut into large florets
- 6 ½ teaspoons extra virgin olive oil, divided
- Pepper
- 2 small avocados

For the chips

- 1 Flatout gluten free flatbread
- 1 teaspoon extra virgin olive oil
- 1 teaspoon lemon zest, packed
- ½ teaspoon garlic salt

For the dressing

- ¼ cup tahini
- ¼ cup cilantro, roughly chopped
- 2 tablespoons mint, chopped
- 2 tablespoons jalapeno, chopped (seeds removed)
- 2 tablespoons water
- 4 teaspoons agave
- 4 teaspoons fresh lemon juice
- ¼ teaspoon salt
- Fresh lemon juice, for garnish

Preparation

i. Remove the grill basket and prepare the grill by heating it to high levels.

ii. Place the half-length sliced potatoes in a large pot, add cold water and salt then boil on high heat. When they start boiling, you can lower the heat to medium level and let them cook for some time until they are tender but not overcooked. The cooking should be about 12 to 15 minutes before draining and setting them aside.

iii. Take the zucchini and slice them into half-width before slicing each half into stick shapes. Add them into a large bowl, pour 2 teaspoons of oil, a pinch of salt and pepper. Place aside, take another bowl, and do the same for the cauliflower.

iv. Place the grill in place, spray with cooking oil and place the cauliflower and zucchini sticks on the grill to cook. The cauliflower should be stirred while cooking, and the zucchini stick can stay in place until one side is charred before flipping and repeating the same on the other side (each side will be cooked within 3 minutes). Allow the cauliflower to cook for some extra minutes after the zucchini are done then remove from the cooker.

v. Embark on the cooled potatoes and slice them into sticks and toss them with 2 teaspoons of oil and some salt. Take the avocado and slice into half, remove the seed and brush the remaining oil on them then sprinkle salt and pepper.

vi. Place both avocado and the sweet potatoes on the grill making sure that the cut side on the avocados is on the grill. Cook each side of the potatoes for about 2 minutes where they will be charred and make sure that the avocados are not burning then remove from the grill.

vii. Take the Flatout and rub with one teaspoon of oil, lemon zest, garlic, and salt. Make sure they are well rubbed on it and then place on the grill and cook for 1 minute on each side.

viii. Using a food processor, place the dressing ingredients, excluding the fresh lemon juice and blend them until they are smooth and creamy.

ix. Peel the avocados then you can serve all the ingredients in bowls then use the lemon juice over the meal and salt to taste if necessary. Also, distribute the grilled Flatout into the bowls equally and enjoy your meal as a main meal of the day.

https://www.foodfaithfitness.com/tahini-grilled-avocado-cauliflower-and-sweet-potato-power-bowl/

LAMB SLOW COOKED & WHITE BEANS STEW

Nutrition

Servings 4

Calorie 461

Carbohydrate 33.4g

Protein 27.5g

Fat 24.2g

Fiber 8.4g

Sugar 9.8g

Ingredients

- 1 tablespoon olive oil
- 350g lamb, diced shoulder
- 2 rashers smoked streaky bacon, roughly chopped
- 2 onions, chopped
- 1 celery stalk, chopped
- 1 carrot, diced
- 2 cloves garlic, roughly chopped
- 1 teaspoon fennel seeds
- 2 red skinned potatoes, peeled and diced
- 400g can white beans, drained and rinsed
- 2 tablespoon tomato puree
- 500ml lamb stock
- 260g spinach

Preparation

i. Heat the saucepan and cook the lamb, bacon, celery, and onions; for five minutes. When they turn brown, add the garlic and fennel then continue cooking for another 1 minute.

ii. Add into the meal the potatoes, beans, puree, and the stock then cover to cook for 50 minutes so that the lamb is tender enough.

iii. Take the spinach and add then stir and allow them to cook for another 1 to 2 minutes before turning off the cooker.

iv. Serve in bowls and enjoy for dinner.

https://www.waitrose.com/content/waitrose/en/home/recipes/recipe_directory/s/slow-cooked-lambandwhitebeanstew.html

LEAN CHICKEN BURGER

Nutrition

Servings 4

Calorie 238

Carbohydrate 11.5g

Protein 28.8g

Fat 7.8g

Cholesterol 110mg

Fiber 0.8g

Sugar 1g

Ingredients

- 1 pound extra-lean ground chicken
- ½ cup Italian seasoned bread crumbs, divided
- ½ small onion, finely grated
- 1 egg
- 2 cloves garlic, minced
- Salt and black pepper (grounded), to taste
- 2 teaspoons olive oil

Preparation

i. Take the grounded chicken, divided bread crumbs, onion and egg then spice them with garlic, salt, and pepper and mix inside a bowl. Take the mixture and start scooping in your moisten hand every 2 tablespoons at a time and make flat and oval patties.

ii. Take the remaining bread crumbs and spread it over a shallow dish. Roll the patties gently on the crumbs to form a coat.

iii. Pour the olive oil in a skillet and heat it over the cooker at medium-high heat.

iv. Transfer the patties into the hot oil and cook one side for about 5 to 6 minutes. Carefully flip them over then continue cooking the other side for another 3 to 4 minutes. Both sides should be brown before removing from the pan.

v. When ready, serve them with some mashed potatoes and salad of choice on the side. You can also use bread rolls and insert the burgers with a salad of your choice and lettuce.

https://www.allrecipes.com/recipe/232375/natashas-chicken-burgers/

GOURMET MUSHROOM RISOTTO

Nutrition

Servings 6

Calories 431

Fat 16.6g

Carbohydrates 56.6g

Fiber 2.7g

Sugars 4g

Protein 11.3g

Cholesterol 29mg

Ingredients

- 6 cups chicken broth, divided
- 3 tablespoons olive oil, divided
- 1 pound Portobello mushroom, sliced thinly
- 1 pound white mushroom, sliced thinly
- 2 shallots, diced
- 1 ½ cups Arborio rice
- ½ cup dry white wine
- Seas salt to taste
- Freshly grounded black pepper to taste
- 3 tablespoons finely chopped chives
- 4 tablespoons butter
- 1/3 cup freshly grated parmesan cheese

Preparation

i. Take the saucepan and place it on a low heat then warm the broth on it.

ii. On another pan, heat 2 spoons of olive oil on medium-high heat. Stir fry the mushrooms taking care to cook them for about 3 minutes then remove their liquid and lay them aside.

iii. On another skillet, add the remaining olive oil and cook the shallots making sure you still well then add rice and cook to coat with the oil for few minutes. Wait until the rice takes a pale golden look before adding the wine then preparing for the wine to absorb.

iv. Take ½ cup of the broth and add to the rice and cook while stirring until it absorbs and repeat the process at a time. In the end, you will have an al dente rice which is achievable in about 20 minutes.

v. Take the skillet off the heater and add the mushrooms then take the butter, chives, parmesan, and salt plus pepper to taste and stir them with the meal.

vi. Serve the meal into six equal portions.

https://www.allrecipes.com/recipe/85389/gourmet-mushroom-risotto/

ASPARAGUS WITH LEMON-GARLIC SAUCE

Nutrition

Servings 6

Calories 129

Fat 10g

Carbohydrates 9g

Protein 2g

Ingredients

- ¼ cups butter
- 2 cloves garlic, sliced thinly
- 1 lemon, juiced
- 2 bunches asparagus, washed
- 1 tablespoon olive oil
- Salt and powder black pepper to taste

Preparation

i.   Place a saucepan on a medium heated cooker then heat the butter and garlic.

ii. Once you see that the garlic is bubbling, lower the heat and let them continue cooking avoiding them to turn brown.

iii. Take the lemon juice and add to the saucepan making sure that the heat is now turned off.

iv. Now use a grill pan over medium-high heat to toss the asparagus having added some olive oil. Grill them for 2 to 3 minutes so that to attain the tenderness and yet crispy nature.

v.   Transfer the asparagus to a baking dish where you will strain the lemon-garlic butter over.

vi. Use salt and pepper to season then toss for them to combine well before serving as a sider for any meat meal.

https://www.thespruceeats.com/grilled-asparagus-lemon-garlic-butter-recipe-101870

GARLIC GREEN BEANS & PORTOBELLOS WITH PARMESAN

Nutrition

Servings 8

Calories 66

Fat 3g

Cholesterol 2mg

Carbohydrates 5g

Fiber 1g

Sugar 2g

Protein 2g

Ingredients

- 2 tablespoons vegetable oil (or ghee)
- 4 Portobello mushrooms, thickly sliced without gills
- 4 cups green beans, snapped
- 5 garlic cloves, minced
- ¼ cup parmesan, finely grated
- Kosher salt and grounded black pepper, to taste

Preparation

i. Place a large pot on the cooker and add the water and heat to boiling then put the beans and cook for about 2 minutes before draining the water.

ii. Heat the oil in a skillet when the heat is at a high level and add the sliced mushroom cooking while occasionally stirring for about 8 minutes, or turns brown. (The mushrooms becomes brown once all their water has evaporated).

iii. Turn the heat lower to medium level and add the boiled beans then the garlic and cook while stirring at the same time season with the salt and the pepper. The cooking should be for 2 minutes and stirring continuously before removing.

iv. Serve the meal on the plates and top with the cheese by sprinkling on the top.

https://www.thewickednoodle.com/green-beans-portobellos/

SOY SAUCE GLAZED MUSHROOMS

Nutrition

Servings 2

Calories 135

Fat 11.9g

Carbohydrate 5.4g

Protein 4.2g

Cholesterol 31mg

Sugars 2g

Fiber 1.4g

Ingredients

- 2 tablespoons butter
- 8 ounces of white mushrooms, sliced
- 2 cloves garlic, minced
- 2 teaspoons soy sauce
- Grounded black pepper to taste

Preparation

i. Switch on the cooker to medium-high then place a skillet and add the mushrooms. Cook while stirring so as they become softened and loses their liquid. About five minutes will be enough.

ii. Add to it the garlic and stir fry for another 1 minutes then you can add the soy sauce. Cook with the sauce for another four minutes or until the liquid has completely evaporated.

iii. Remove the skillet and switch off the heat.

iv. You can serve over any meat of your choice.

https://www.allrecipes.com/recipe/58112/mushrooms-with-a-soy-sauce-glaze/

SESAME GINGER MISO CUCUMBER SALAD

Nutrition

Servings 4

Calories 287

Carbohydrates 39g

Fiber 10g

Sugar 17g

Protein 15g

Cholesterol 11mg

Fat 10g

Ingredients

Salad

- 2 large English cucumbers
- 1 ½ cups frozen shelled edamame, defrosted
- 2 medium carrots, julienned
- 1 tablespoon toasted white and black sesame seeds
- 1 sheet of nori

Dressing

- 2 ½ tablespoons white miso
- 1 ½ tablespoons hot water
- 2 tablespoons rice vinegar
- 1 ½ tablespoon grated ginger, peeled
- 1 tablespoon honey or maple syrup
- 1 ½ tablespoon sesame oil
- 2 teaspoons lemon juice, lemon extract
- ½ teaspoon tamari sauce

Preparation

i. Take the cucumbers and prepare larger noodles using a spiralizer fit with a wider blade. Make sure you sprit the noodles by cutting every 12 to 15 inches length.

ii. Place the prepared noodles into a large bowl and put the Edamame and carrots and toss them together.

iii. In a different and smaller bowl, whisk the water and miso together until they are smooth. Later add the rest of the dressing ingredients and continue mixing and make sure you add the taste you prefer; whether saltier or sweeter.

iv. Put the vegetables and the dressing together and continue tossing to mix thoroughly.

v. Take some sesame seeds and sprinkle on the top as you desire and serve together with some slices of Nori.

https://www.snixykitchen.com/sesame-ginger-miso-cucumber-salad/

CHICKEN, BURGHUL & POMEGRANATE SALADNUTRITION

Servings 1
Calorie 493
Carbohydrate 49.5g
Protein 34.5g
Fat 15g
Fiber 10.8g
Salt 0.2g

Ingredients

- 50g bulgar heat
- 20g sultanas
- Saffron
- 1 chicken breast skinless
- Oil
- 1 teaspoon pomegranate molasses, plus more
- ½ small red onion, finely diced
- 1 tablespoon almonds flaked, toasted
- 1 teaspoon red wine vinegar
- A handful rocket

Preparation

i. Prepare an oven and take it to 200 degrees Fahrenheit. Place a pan with water to boiling point before adding the wheat covered with Clingfilm then allow them to absorb for about 10 to 15 minutes. Drain the water afterward and set aside. Take the sultana and saffron into a bowl and pour a tablespoon of hot water then mix.

ii. Take a teaspoon of oil and apply on the chicken before drizzling the molasses and seasoning then cook by roasting for 20 to 30 minutes so that it is thoroughly done.

iii. Add into the cooking meal the onions, almonds, vinegar and bulgar then season to your taste. Toss the sultanas plus their juice and season as per your preference/

iv.   Use the rocket and salad to serve with slices of chicken as you use some pomegranate molasses to drizzle.

https://www.olivemagazine.com/recipes/healthy/pomegranate-roasted-chicken-with-bulgar-wheat-salad/

www.ingramcontent.com/pod-product-compliance
Lightning Source LLC
Chambersburg PA
CBHW020613220526
45463CB00006B/2577